Be Healed In Your Veins & Arteries

Stellah Mupanduki

Genre: Health, Self-Help, Body, Soul and Spirit, Christian Living, Books of Ministry.

Target Audience: All people: Male and female. Terminally ill people. Depressed people. Mentally ill people. Counselling groups. Synonymous groups. Outreach groups. Schools and Universities. Churches. Hospitals.

About the Book: Be Healed In Your Veins &Arteries.

Be Healed in Your Veins and Arteries is an anointed, powerful book that heals veins and arteries. It touches the heart, and blood vessels with a powerful and healing, cleansing and protection from terminal illness, rare and all "incurable" diseases of the heart and veins and arteries. Read this book and be cleansed, healed and protected from dreaded diseases of the veins and arteries. Be protected in your heart and body and blood vessels.

Chapter

1. Be healed In Your Veins & Arteries

Dedicated.

To the whole world for the healing and protection of hearts

For the love of those who are suffering from heart diseases

To all those who seek true healing from God Almighty

To all those seeking personal healing and salvation

For the healing of the world that God created

To those who love to be have blessed hearts

For the peace of those hearts troubled

To the church and all families of God

For salvation of terminally ill people

For internal healing of the body

For the blessing of whole body

For sound Internal Organs.

To my children

Favour of God

Sound Family.

Romans 8:29-30

"For those God foreknew he also predestined to be conformed to the likeness of his Son, that he might be the firstborn among many brothers. And those he predestined, he also called; those he called, he also justified; and those he justified, he also glorified."

Acknowledgement

Through Jesus Christ, Son of the Living God...These extraordinary books were written in the Truthful Leading, Healing, Guiding, Comforting, Pouring and Teaching of the Holy Spirit for the healing benefit of his people. No person or medical professional being, made any contribution to the writing of these books except the Holy Spirit himself using the author. He is the teacher and the healer and author of all mankind and creation. These books bring powerful intercession for healing before God on your behalf and allow you to communicate with the highest power in your life in a very free, calm, reassuring and fearless way. God is our best friend and Father full of love. As you read, you should smell the rich scent of the blood of Jesus Christ and as you close your eyes, you should see the cross where our Saviour died as a sign of your salvation.

Psalm 147:1 "Praise the LORD. How good it is to sing praises to our God, how pleasant and fitting to praise him."

For the Healing of Terminal illness, rare and incurable diseases books;

All in all, these powerful holy books are innovatively invented by God Almighty himself for the Healing of Terminal illness, rare and incurable diseases...they bring cleansing and protection to any person in this world. They take away brokenness, disgrace and hopelessness...they build up and they reconstruct...they mould everything...there is amazing Health Care and longevity...there are miracles and wonders...there is goodness and strength. Hallelujah! These books bring salvation through unique healing and peace to the people and all nations and all creation...They boost up every economy of every nation in this whole world. There is the solid truth about everything, there is divine love and compassion of God Almighty for his creation and people...Families are blessed with righteousness, blissful love, established stability, grace and peace from God Almighty in the name of Jesus Christ...There is blissful beauty, marvellous growth, joy and happiness... In creating these books, God Almighty, the Holy Spirit uses the life of a woman who is his vessel of his presence, glory and honour in order to bring salvation and personal liberty and strength to all mankind and their surrounding...This whole world should praise and honour the Holy Spirit of the Sovereign God in all humbleness for his love and mercy...Hallelujah! "Thank you Father God...Thank you my Lord Jesus Christ...Thank you Holy Spirit...triune God...three in One...One in Three. I honour you...Maker of heaven and earth and everything in it...I love you from Everlasting to Everlasting...Amen"

The Lord God Almighty said this to me; "Put these words of healing on paper as books...write them down so that my people will be healed and find peace in their lives and live longer..." And so this extra special gift of healing that is normally experienced on crusades is anointed and put on paper, written for the benefit of mankind and spread through the long and lasting, widespread book publishing industry. Man is mortal and I am a person who will come to cease existence from this world but the Word of God will remain for generations and generations and generations for the healing and salvation of mankind. Yeah...My time on earth as a vessel of God`s glory and honour will come to an end when I am very, very, very old and grey and strong and

powerful in the Lord…and I will go in his powerful glory.
But the world will remain with all these unique books written
by the Holy Spirit and operating in the healing, cleansing,
protecting and saving presence of God himself.

• *"Nothing in these books should be added or subtracted…"*
Says the Lord God Almighty, who created heaven and earth.

NB: These Anointed and Sacred Healing For Terminal
Illness, Rare and all Incurable diseases books will bring true,
inclusive, holy, uniquely unique, pure, peaceful, stable,
happy, exciting, interesting, gripping, comforting,
stabilizing and established, complete and permanent healing
into your whole life and your family, your country, your
continent and the whole world.

• Because of the Feeling of the Wounds of Christ, the Voice
and the Sacred Heart of Christ in me; I am Uniquely
Unique. Hallelujah.

Guidance

About Stellah Mupanduki

Healing For Terminal Illness Ministry:

Stellah Mupanduki of Jesus Christ...is a Charismatic Pentecostal Christian/*Interdenominational*... an Author, and has a miracle working Ministry for Spiritual healing for Terminal illness founded through the anointing power of the Holy Spirit. The essential principle she gives emphasis to and finds viable through her work is that there is hope for terminal illness and it is healed through Jesus Christ our Saviour. There is Hope for the hopeless. The Ministry is founded through a direct calling from God himself and operates in that realm of the Holy Spirit. She holds a Bachelors of Arts degree from the University of Zimbabwe(UZ) and a BCom (Specialising in Risk Management) from the University of South Africa (UNISA) and a Computer Business Application Specialist (Microsoft Office Certification) diploma. She has a liberating specific healing ministry that takes away desolation and death from those who can no longer be helped in the medical field. God is the answer when we are completely devoid of any ideas to help the hopeless. **The Ministry takes away the grave, death sentences, fear, helplessness, disappointments and humiliation of untimely death by removing and eradicating diseases called terminal illness, rare and incurable diseases. Such diseases are now termed as historical because they are being removed and completely eradicated in the name of Jesus Christ.....For generations and generations until the ends of time, they are no more. Consider it done and finished. You do not have to worry anymore for *the Lord says this in the book of Isaiah 44: 24,26* "*I am the Lord, your saviour; I am the one who created you.***

*I am the **LORD**, the Creator of all things. I alone stretched out the heavens; when I made the earth, no one helped me…...But when my servant makes a prediction, when I sent a messenger to reveal my plans, I make those plans and predictions come true." **GNB…***

The Holy Spirit/Feeling of the wounds of Christ/Sacred heart is the greatest and unique person who has enabled the founder to operate and to write nervous system touching and healing, cleansing and protecting books that bring healing help to the hopeless and helpless depending upon his work and guidance that reaches out to the world. There is that holy divine purity in her work. And there is compassion and love for human life in these books. The love of music has helped her connect with the higher power of God that touches people and bring change in their lives. To be generous and kind at heart is a gift from God. Triune God as in God the Father, Son and the Holy Spirit. Three in One and One in three…Being used by God has made her realise how far-reaching God`s love is through Jesus Christ our Saviour. For a person who is terminally ill, these books should be read on their own and should not be mixed with any other works of another person, great or unknown (small). **Healing For Terminal Illness: Golgotha Hallelujah! Thank you Jesus Christ! Thank you Holy Spirit my Father, Jehovah Raphe, Almighty God, Holy One, Sovereign I AM…Hallelujah!**

Other than life troubles in various areas of a person`s life, the Stellah Mupanduki books and personal presence give to the world a radical powerful healing, cleansing and protection from terminal illnesses, rare diseases and all controlling, incurable diseases. For Instance; **Cancers like; brain cancer, skin cancer, renal cancer, lung cancer, leukemia(Blood cancer), bladder cancer, uterine cancer, breast cancer, ovarian cancer,** cervical cancer, prostate cancer, Oesophageal cancer, colorectal cancer, bile duct cancer, liver cancer, cancer of the pancreas, spleen cancer, bone cancer, bone marrow cancer, jaw cancer, cancer of the mouth, colon cancer, stomach cancer, cancer of the lymph nodes, throat cancer, cancer of the internal organs etc. ... for body, soul and mind healing, brain tumours, body tumours, Lung diseases, Chronic body pain...Alzheimer's, Multiple Sclerosis, Coma, Leukemia, Heart diseases, Heart attacks and Stroke, High and low blood pressure, Arthritis, Epilepsy, Parkinson, HIV/AIDS, Lupus, brain diseases, Nervous system, internal organs, Progeria (Rare diseases), Asthma, Cystic fibrosis, Bones and marrow. The backbone, the Spine, obese, elephantiasis, Cholesterol, thrombosis, Diabetes, chronic stomach diseases, chronic incontinence, ulcers, anorexia, chronic depression, brain disorder-mental, neurological diseases...Cerebral Palsy, Sickle Cell Disease, leprosy...migraine, SIDS, skin diseases, osteoporosis, thyroid, Cysts, fibroids, veins and arteries, blood and genetic disorders, Dyslexia, ADD, Autism, down syndrome, sepsis, viruses, curses, allergies, eye diseases, mouth and ears: Speech problems, panic attacks, Cataracts, deaf and dumb, rare and incurable diseases, Barrenness: Womb healing; in matters of illness of the womb. Conceiving and protection from miscarriages........Substance abuse: Drug addiction...The Holy Spirit touches your body with his healing flow and heals all diseases in his supernatural way and ability....My duty is to take everything the Holy Spirit of a Sovereign God is giving and I put it in writing for you to be healed and to fellowship with him...Hallelujah! Healing! Salvation!

Publisher Bookstore Link:

<u>NB</u>: These Godly Invented Nerve Touching Healing Lullabies titles above took Me & the Holy Spirit, 8years of writing and editing. I was taught everything by the Holy Spirit of the Sovereign God himself. When he gave me the direction and command to publish these Healing lullabies books, he also gave me a dream of many stars in the dark sky; meaning, all people of all nations will be touched and healed in his name and power through these holy healing books....<u>Just as the 10 Commandments were given to Moses by God Almighty; these healing lullabies are given directly from God Almighty to a woman, for the healing of nations and all people in the name of Jesus Christ</u>...the Cross...You have to look at the cross and be healed in this era that we are living in this land of the living....<u>God does not change</u> and <u>will never change nor</u> matter what is done or what happens...The Spirit of God will always reveal himself in what he says and does.

Isaiah 40:3-5, "A voice of one calling; "In the desert prepare the way for the LORD; make straight in the wilderness a highway for our God. Every valley shall be raised up, every mountain and hill made low; the rough road shall become level, the rugged places a plain. And the glory of the LORD will be revealed and all mankind will see it. For the mouth of the LORD has spoken."" NIV Bible.

<u>**Advice on how to Read the Lullabies Healing books invented by God Almighty for all his children on earth**</u>: And to all my readers, the presence of the Spirit of the Sovereign God is marked and felt by feelings felt during the process of reading.

Hence you have to read them in your own private time when you are alone. Go into your reading room, your place of comfort and read as you lie down on your sofa, or just go into your bedroom, your solace, close your doors, lie down on your bed and just read and be touched in a deep and healing way by the Holy Spirit of a Sovereign God Almighty. Be in an undisturbed environment and enjoy the presence of God Almighty as you read and fellowship with him. Its all about you and the Holy Spirit.

And the *__Healing Notes To the Readers of My Work is__: The uniquely unique powerful presence of God you feel as you read my work is also the presence of the Holy Spirit you will feel when I am public speaking, teaching and ministering in your presence. And God makes me feel you as he heals you by touching my body with the healing touch you are receiving from him...There is nothing that God does not reveal to me his vessel of his presence, glory and honour...If he is healing breast cancer, he reveals to me...if he is touching strokes, he touches even one side of my body to show that someone with a right side stroke or left side stroke is being healed...he touches from the top of the head to the sole of the foot of that affected side...When he touches the brain, he reveals...When he goes to the heart, he shows this to me as well. He reveals his stabilising stability....When he touches the nerves and nervous system, he greatly touches me as well...he shows me...When he touches the lungs, he reveals...when he goes to the womb and all reproductive organs, he reveals...he reveals prostate cancer being healed by touching my abdomen as well...When he touches the spine, he reveals to me as well...He tells me who he is healing and what he is healing....And when he touches you from the top of your head with a strong grip and all the way to the soles of your feet, he also mercifully touches me*

*with that healing flow you are receiving that feels like goose
bumps on your skin...He touches your inner most being as
well as my own inner-most being for me to be able to write
and say this to you...Hence the recipient and the vessel of
God have the same touch from the Almighty One for his
glorification...We are all One in Christ, you and me...Hence I
am able to praise him for you and me as well.*

*Therefore, read these books without mixing them with any
other person's works except the Holy Bible itself, in its
purity, that was breathed by the Spirit of God Almighty to
the vessels who wrote it in days of old....No one in today's
age should ever add or subtract anything in the Holy Bible
by writing in it or commenting in it because commenting
between lines or paragraphs in the bible will cause spiritual
warfare to the reader no matter how powerful and well-
known an author is...Respect the Holy Bible. Read the bible
in its original form without any intrusion from people who
write in it...This is not being selfish but helping you readers
to receive pure and holy maximum healing from the Holy
Spirit as he commands and speaks to your hearts in his
purity, and for you to be able to give him the glory he
deserves in order for him to pour himself out to the nations
and people for more blessings...Benefit from the wounds of
Christ and receive pure healing. This will work for you
because there is true, complete and permanent healing from
God Almighty, Maker of heaven and earth...Put 100% trust in
God alone and you will be set free in permanent
completeness... The Holy Spirit, the Spirit of the Sovereign
God has poured out for you in order to be set free from all
strongholds and I have put in writing everything he gave to
you in these books.....Overcome the spirit of terminal illness,*

rare and incurable diseases...Purity! Safety! Healing! Protection! Hallelujah!

And the word of encouragement and truth I give about the Stellah Mupanduki books is that they should also be read to those who cannot read for themselves **because of illness**, or because of the fact that they are **babies** and those who are in a **Coma**...And to my **able readers**...As you read and absorb the prophetic healing words in these nervous system touching healing handiwork...you will experience the powerful supernatural healing presence of the Holy Spirit touching and healing your body inside and out. You will feel him on your skin and inside you...The healing Word in these books is about the *reader* and the Holy Spirit, it is about *you* and The Holy Spirit.

Holy...Holy: As you read these books, when you feel compelled to breathe his breath in ...do so...inhale his healing breath...make long and strong inhaling pulls...you will feel touched from the top of your head all the way to the soles of your feet...you will be touched on areas of your body that are troubling you...breathe in strongly and long and be healed. You will feel him touching you from the inside as you make these strong inhaling pulls...*Praise the Lord:* When you come on instances where the blood of Christ is mentioned and you start to choke, and cough or feel it in your throat, do not stop reading...keep going because anything bad in your body will be removed...keep reading do not be scared because you will be doing the right thing for your salvation...You are freed!

Hallelujah: When you feel your whole body filled with a soothing and cool wind...do not panic for God will be healing you in completeness....so let it be...*Holy:* When you feel compelled to be still and know he is God...go ahead and honour him through this anointing time of healing taking place in your body, put your book down and be quiet and still in body, just let go of yourself and allow the Holy Spirit of God to take control of your body, soul and spirit... *Glory:* When you feel compelled to keep reading...do so, keep absorbing because the Spirit of the Sovereign Lord is upon you helping you in this powerful healing journey. *Hosanna:* When you feel overwhelmed with his love and healing in your life and are compelled to praise Him and sing with Him and glorify His Name ...do so and be holy in his holiness...take the song that is put into your heart by the Holy Spirit himself and sing it in the way you love...*Praise the Lord!*

Thank you Lord: When you feel compelled to say out everything in your heart to him, do so, pour out all your feelings, your needs, your fears, your worries, your anger, your hurting, your loneliness in this time of affliction, say out whatever it is that you are going through when you feel compelled to do so...remove the death feeling from your soul ...*glory...glory...glory*...give everything to the Holy Spirit until you feel emptied of all burdens and your body, soul and mind feel light and relieved from burdens...just pour out your crying heart to the Lord God Almighty and he will answer you and heal you and comfort you in truth and in spirit....God Almighty will take away all rough patches in your life...He will remove all trials and all tribulations for you...the Lord who is your God will level your mountain...he will take all those burdens from you and you will never feel them or experience them in your life, and in your body, soul and mind again...Your life will be fine...the Lord Almighty will protect you from the negative throws of life...the Lord Almighty, the Sovereign I AM will remove all weakness from your life and you will truthfully overcome in great peace...there is healing for you...*Glory be to God Almighty.*

Hosanna: When there is a forceful continuous yawning, do not fight against the yawning...allow the yawning to go on until the Holy Spirit stops and you will feel very liberated and light in body...this is your key to your salvation...there is release of all evil and tension...the heavy burdens will be removed...you will feel the yawning strength and beauty in the healing that you will be experiencing...If you are reading to a child/baby; when they start this yawning process, **shout Hosanna to God Almighty** for true and permanent healing will be taking place, your child/baby will live ... *Cherubim... Cherubim... Hallelujah!*

Thank you Lord. When you feel warm in particular parts of your body, be happy...be relieved because God Almighty in the name of Jesus Christ is healing that part of your body...Finally when you feel his warmth wrapping around you and you need to sleep...put your book aside and sleep and feel nurtured as the healing flow of God Almighty spreads in your body in quietness...*Holy...holy...holy God Almighty: When you feel all weak in your body and you cannot do anything, and it feels like you are bound from doing anything for yourself...do not worry at all, it is all fine because God Almighty, will be breaking the illness and all evil for you......stay put, allow that weak and broken feeling in your body to prevail until you feel strong again. The Lord will give you that strength...you will be fine...you will regain strength!*

Glory be to God Almighty...Salvation... Hallelujah: As you sleep, in the name of Jesus Christ, you will hear the helping voice of the Holy Spirit interceding on your behalf in your dreams...you will hear him praying for you and with you in his name...you will find yourself praying as you sleep dreaming dreams of your life and you wake up to realise that you were really praying facing a particular situation in your life e.g., dreams of someone in all black chasing you with a weapon, or some form of war where your life is at risk, or someone advancing at you in order to attack, or just being sick and helpless and in all this you overcome because you become very strong and vehement in prayer facing the warring situation...The Holy Spirit is living and active, emphatic and triumphant for you....You win...You will definitely love the Holy Spirit, the helper of your life, the Sovereign I AM...*Holy...holy...holy*! You will have wonderful healing and overcoming dreams of light, growth, the cross, water, the sun and moon and many more salvation dreams as given by the Holy Spirit himself to you...You will be renewed and refreshed when you wake up. You will regain strength and be filled with smiles because of the protecting and assuring divine helping presence of our merciful and forgiving God Almighty...*Glory!*

So as you finish reading these holy and sacred healing books, you will rise up because you will be set free. Jesus Christ came for you to be healed and be set free from all strongholds of life. **Terminal illness, rare and incurable diseases can no longer scare you or make you live a fearful and uncertain life because there is healing in the name of Jesus Christ. Healing! Cleansing! Salvation! Protection! Joy! Hallelujah!**

Through his Name and blood, no life is left unchanged. God is merciful and loving to all. He is the Power in your life. **And His healing flow in your body and his truthful presence will set you free as you read these sacred and holy books.** Do not be afraid...read and find inner peace...Do not succumb to discouragement, troubles and death... There is healing coming from God Almighty to you... There is no one like our God...*Beautiful Hallelujah! Hosanna! Amen.*

Powered by the Finger of God...Holy Spirit...Living and

Active. (Guidance on Reading is put in every new manuscript produced)

Isaiah 44: 23 "Shout for joy, you heavens. Shout, deep places of the earth! Shout for joy, mountains and every tree of the forest! The LORD has shown his greatness by saving his people Israel" GNB.

<u>Chapter 1</u>

Be Healed In Your Veins And Arteries

Psalm 37:5

"Commit your way to the LORD; trust him."

* May the Lord give strength and success to the blood circulating system. May the Lord make a good and sound way for blood flow in the veins and arteries...**Be healed in all your veins and arteries**...be healed from the top of your head and all the way to the soles of your feet...**be healed from illness of the heart, veins and arteries**...be well in your blood...be healthy in your heart, veins and arteries...be healed in that wonderful name of the Lord Jesus Christ...

May the good Lord keep and make perfect the natural order of things in your body system and heart...Be healed in your heart and body... be healed in veins and arteries...be well in the blood that flow in your veins and arteries...**Be healed from blood cancer**...be well in your veins and arteries...be strong in your veins and arteries...be purified in the blood that flow in your veins and arteries...**be healed from terminal illness of the heart, veins, arteries and blood**...be purified in the blood that flow in your veins and arteries...**be well in**

the heart that pumps blood in your body through blood vessels…be living and active in your heart, veins and arteries…be strong and well in your body, heart, veins and arteries…**be healed through the healing power of God Almighty**…be healed in your veins and arteries…**be healed from illness of the veins and arteries**…be healed in your heart…be healed in that powerful name of the Lord Jesus Christ…May the good Lord immerse your heart in the saving and protecting blood of the Lord Jesus Christ…may his healing power and presence remove all illness, clots and bad cholesterol from the blood that flow in your veins and arteries…Be healed in your heart…Be healed in your veins and arteries…be set free from the spirit of clotting of blood in your veins and arteries…**be set free from the rupture of veins and arteries**…be healed with a good blood circulation…be healed in your veins and arteries…be healed from cancer…be healed from illness of veins and arteries…be healed from illness of the heart…be healed on your skin…be beautiful on your skin…be set free from blood diseases…be healed with a good flow of blood in your veins and arteries…**be healed from constriction of the veins, arteries and the heart**…be relaxed in your heart, veins and arteries…be healthy in your heart, veins and arteries…be healed in your heart…be at peace in the heart…be well in your heart, veins and arteries…be healed with righteous and supernatural peace in your heart…be healed in that wonderful name of the Lord Jesus Christ…May there be goodness and power and beauty in the blood that circulate in your veins and arteries…**May the Lord God Almighty make everything right for you in your physical heart**…Be healed with vigour in every part of the heart…be healed with permanent healing in your heart…Be healed from pain in the heart…be healed from weakness of the heart…be healed in all your heart muscles…be strong in your heart muscles…be well in your heart…be healed from struggling in the heart…**be healed from illness of the heart**…be strong in your heart…be able to endure…be powerful in your heart…be healthy in your heart…be healed through the powerful power of the Lord God Almighty…Be healed from illness of the heart…**be set free from a heart disorder**…be healed in that powerful name of the Lord Jesus Christ…May the Lord in his compassion bless the body with a good and healthy heart bit. Be healed in your heart that pumps blood in your body…**be healed in veins and arteries**…be healed in every chamber of the heart…be healed from illness of the heart…be healed from a heart disease…be healed with a good and healthy heart…be healed through the healing power of God Almighty, who is Maker of heaven and earth…be healed in vigour…be healed with a mighty strength of healing from the Lord God Almighty…be healed in your heart and body…be healed from the top of your head and all the way to the soles of your feet…be protected from the spirit of strokes…be protected in your heart…be sound in the heart…be healed my good friend…be healed in your heart…be healed from all heart diseases…be protected from heart diseases…be healed in every part of your heart…be healed in that powerful and saving name of the Lord Jesus Christ. May the heart live long in good peace from God…be healed in his power that is above all powers…the power of the Lord God Almighty, Maker of heaven and earth.

* **Dear Reader**, dedicate yourself to God Almighty; "Triune God, Holy Father, Holy Jesus Christ, Holy Spirit…you are everything to me…I belong to you alone…Heal my heart and make me strong again. Help me to walk in peace and stability. Raise me from my place of illness. Speak healing words to my heart again and again. Help me up and I will be saved. Bring goodness in my blood and make me live without fear of falling. I love you God Almighty, Maker of heaven and earth. I love you my Lord Jesus Christ. I honour you Holy Spirit. Help me to live and glorify your name every day of my life."

Psalm 81:13-14

"If my people would but listen to me, if Israel would follow my ways, how quickly would I subdue their enemies and turn my hand against their foes!"

* May the good Lord protect and give sound healing to all your heart chambers. May they receive and discharge in goodness. May he remove intrusion from foreign obstacles and substances…Be healed with goodness in your heart chambers…be healed in every cell, be healed in all fluid…**be healed in every heart muscle…be healed in all fibre and tissues**…be healed in the wonderful name of the Lord Jesus Christ…May the Lord God Almighty bring forth a good and viable circulation of blood in the heart and in your body…Be healed in completeness in your heart chambers…be healed in that powerful name of the Lord Jesus Christ…be well in your heart…be healed from the top of your head and all the way to the soles of your feet…be healed on the left side of your body…be healed from the top of your head and all the way to the sole of your left foot…**be healed from paralysis of the left side**…be healed in your heart…be healed with goodness in your heart and body…be able to move well in your body parts…be able to use your hand and leg…be able to walk well…be healed in your body…be healed from stroke…be healed in the wonderful and powerful name of the Lord Jesus Christ…Be healthy in your body…be restored to goodness through the healing power of God Almighty…Be healed in your motor skills…be healed in all your sensory nerves…be able to see…be able to hear…be able to eat and chew…be able to smell and touch and feel…be able to speak…be able to move well

in all your body parts…function well in your body, heart
and mind…be healed from the spirit of paralysis…be
healed in your body…Recover well in your body, heart
and mind…be immersed in that powerful blood of the
Lord Jesus Christ…be revived in your body, heart and
mind…be immersed in the saving and protecting blood
of the Lord Jesus Christ, the Lamb of God who took
away the sins of the world…Be healed in your body…be
healed through the powerful healing power of God
Almighty…be healed with a complete and permanent
reviving healing from God Almighty…be healthy in your
heart and body…be healthy in that wonderful name of
the Lord Jesus Christ…Hallelujah.

Be healed from stroke…be healed from the spirit of
paralysis…**be healed from the right side of your
body**…be healed from the top of your head and all the
way to the sole of your right foot…be healed with a
powerful healing flow of God Almighty…be healed on
the right side of your body…be healed in your sensory
nerves…be healed in all your motor skills…be healed
from paralysis…be able to move your right side of your
body…be healed from stroke…be healed from
paralysis…be able to move your neck…be able to move
your body…be able to move your hands and legs…be
able to feel your body parts…be healed from
paralysis…be well again in your body…be able to
hear…be able to speak…be able to chew and eat…be
able to swallow…**be healed from the spirit of**

paralysis…be well in your mouth…be healed in your jaws…be healed through the healing flow of God Almighty who is Maker of heaven and earth…be healed in every part of the right side of your body…be healed in your heart…be healed in all internal organs…be healed from stroke…be healed in your reproductive organs…**be healed in the veins and arteries…**be healed in the blood that flow in your veins and arteries…be restored to goodness in your body…be revived in every part of your body…Be revived in all sides of your body…be revived on the left side of your body, from the top of your head and all the way to the sole of your feet…be revived on the right side of your body from the top of your head and all the way to the soles of your feet…be healed in every part of your body…be revived in completeness from the top of your head and all the way to the soles of your feet…be able to move your head, and body, from the top of your head and all the way to the soles of your feet…be healed on the neck…be at peace on your neck…have feelings and goodness on the neck…be healed with good movement…be healed in the name of the Lord Jesus Christ…Be able to feel your chest…be in good movement in the chest…be revived in your chest…be healthy in your chest…be healed in that powerful name of the Lord Jesus Christ…be able to have body feeling of your waist and down…be able to feel your waist and own…be able to move your body from the top of your head and all the way to the soles of your feet...be revived in the waist...be revived in the backbone...be revived in the spine...be revived in all your legs and feet...be healed from the spirit of stroke...be healed from the spirit of paralysis...be healed with goodness and good health in your body...be able to walk...be able to use your hands...be able to use your hands and legs...be able to move your body...be able to speak and be heard...be healed in all muscles of the body...be healed in every fibre...be healed in every tissue...be healed in every cell...be healed in all glands...be healed in all body fluid...have ability in your body...be healed in joints and muscles of your body...be healed in your nervous system...be well again in your body...have stability and ability in every part of your body...be healed with a good coordinating body system...be healed in your heart, brain and body...be healed from stroke...be healed from paralysis...be well in your body and spirit...Be fully immersed in the saving and protecting blood of the Lord Jesus Christ...Be protected in your heart...be protected from heart failure...be protected from all heart diseases...be protected in your heart and brain...be protected in your body...be completely protected through the glory of God Almighty...be protected in his living power and mercy...be protected from the top of your head and all the way to the soles of your feet...be protected in that powerful name of the Lord Jesus Christ…Thank you Holy Spirit.

Dear Reader; make a renewal request from God; "Make me humble before you my Lord God Almighty so that it is well with my heart and soul…"

Isaiah 62: 10

"Pass through, pass through the gates! Prepare the way for the people. Build up, build up the highway! Remove the stones. Raise a Banner for the nations."

* May the Lord God Almighty in the name of Jesus Christ, remove all impurities of the blood…**be cleansed in your veins and arteries**…have wonderful movement of blood in your veins and arteries…**be healed from plaque in your veins and arteries**…be cleansed in your heart, veins and arteries…**May the Good Lord Almighty iron out cholesterol**…may he help your veins and arteries to be relaxed and open well for the passing through of blood…may the Lord Almighty cleanse your blood to perfection…may our God who is mighty to save be merciful to you and heal you in the blood, veins and arteries…**may he remove all blood clots and bring goodness to your blood and blood vessels**…may he heal you from all chronic illness of the blood…may the Lord remove bad cholesterol from your heart and body and blood…may the Lord iron it out…may he make your blood to flow smoothly in your veins and arteries…may the Lord touch your blood and purify it…may he breathe in his good healing breath into your blood and give purity and good health all the days of your life…**Be healed from high blood pressure…be healed in the blood that flow in your veins and arteries**…be healed in your heart…be cleansed in your blood…be healed from all diseases and suffering of the blood, veins and arteries…be healed from the spirit of blockage…be healed in your veins and arteries…be healed in every part of your heart…**be healed from chronic illness of the blood**…be set free from the spirit of high blood pressure…be at peace in your heart and brain…be protected from the attacks of high blood pressure…be healed in your blood…**be healed from high blood pressure…be healed from low blood pressure…be healed in your body…be healed in your heart…**be healed through the power of the living God…be healed with vigour in your blood…be purified in your blood…be healed from the spirit of infirmity of the blood…be healed in that wonderful name of the Lord Jesus Christ…Be at peace in the blood that flow in your veins and arteries**…be healed from chronic headaches caused by illness of blood, veins and arteries**……be healed from chronic heart disease…be protected from the spirit of strokes…be saved from the spirit of heart attacks…be strong in your body…be healed in your blood…be healed from the attacks of high blood pressure…it is bound from prevailing…**high blood pressure is removed from your body**…high blood pressure is no more…regain strength in your body…regain strength in your blood…**be cleansed from all impurities of the blood**…be peaceful in the flow of your blood in your veins and arteries…be strong in veins and arteries…**be healed from chronic illness of the heart, veins and arteries**…be healed in your heart…be healed in that wonderful name of the Lord Jesus Christ…Be healed with goodness in your heart…be healed in your blood…**be healed from the spirit of high and low blood pressure…**be healed in your veins and arteries…be healed from heart strokes…be healed from high blood pressure…**be healed in your veins and arteries**…be protected from rapturing of veins and arteries…**be protected from hemorrhoids**…be protected from strokes…be healed from high blood pressure…be healed in your heart and mind…be healed and be protected in your brain…be healed in your body…be strong in your body frame…be stable and normal in your blood…**be healthy in the blood, veins and arteries**…**be healed from the macabre spirit of high and low blood pressure…High and low blood pressure** is cancelled…it is no more…it is removed…it is wiped out of your veins, arteries and body…it has no power in your body, soul and spirit…Hallelujah! Be permanently healed from this chronic illness of the blood...it is cut-off from rising...it is overpowered...it is eradicated from your blood, veins and arteries...**be at peace in your body, heart, blood, veins and arteries**...be immersed in the saving blood of the Lord Jesus Christ...Be healed from the top of your head all the way to the soles of your feet...be healed in every cell, in every fibre, in all fluid, in all glands, joints an marrow...be healed and be strong in your body, veins and arteries...be healthy in your heart...be healthy in every part of your heart...be healed from illness of the heart, blood, veins and arteries...be protected from heart failure...be healed in your body...be healed through the mighty power of God Almighty, who is Maker of heaven and earth...be healthy in the wonderful and saving name of the Lord Jesus Christ. Be healed in your brain...be healed and be protected in your motor skills...be protected in all your sensory nerves...be protected in your sense of feeling...be protected in your sense of smell...**be protected in your eye sight**...be protected in your hearing...be healed in your brain...be healed from strokes...be healed from the spirit of heart attacks...be protected from strokes...be protected from heart attacks...be healed from the top of your head and all the way to the soles of your feet...be healed through the healing power of God Almighty who is Maker of heaven and earth, seas and oceans, rolling rivers and lakes and everything in them...be healed through his mercy and love...be healthy in your body...be at peace in all your nerves…be healed in your blood…be healed in your heart…**be set free from heart attacks…be set free from heart failure**…**be healed from high and low blood pressure**…be cleansed in your blood…be protected in your heart and mind…be immersed in the saving and protecting blood of the Lord Jesus Christ, the Lamb of God who took away the sins of the world…be healed in that powerful name of the Lord Jesus Christ…Thank you Holy Spirit, you are God and you are good…I love you Lord…May your name be blessed forever and ever…Hallelujah! Amen!

Deuteronomy 11:13-15

"So if you faithfully obey the commands I am giving you today- to love the LORD your God and to serve him with all your heart and with all your soul- then I will send rain on your land in its season, both autumn and spring rains, so that you may gather in your grain, new wine and oil. I will provide grass in the fields for your cattle, and you will eat and be satisfied.""

* Be healed in your heart…be healed through the powerful power of God Almighty who created you…be healed in every part of your heart…**be completely healed in every valve…be healed in every artery…be healed from illness**…be healed from brokenness in the physical heart.be healed in every artery…be healed in all muscles of the heart…be healed from illness of the

heart…be strong in the heart…Be healed in all heart chambers…be healed with goodness…be set free from illness of the heart…be healed through the healing flow of God Almighty, who is Maker of heaven and earth, seas and oceans, rolling rivers and lakes and everything in them…be healed in his strength and love…be healed in your heart…**be healed in every vein…be healed in every artery…be healed in every valve**…be healed in every fibre and every muscle of the heart…be healed in all tissues of the heart…be healed in all fluid…be healed in every cell…be healed in the blood that flows in your body…be healed from illness of the heart…be saved from failure of the heart…be immersed in the saving and protecting blood of the Lord Jesus Christ, the Lamb of God who took away the sins of the world…Be healthy in the name of the Lord…maintain your bodies…have life…live your normal lives in the name of the Lord Jesus Christ…Be happy and contented in his glorious presence. May the good Lord bring happiness to your heart. **Be healed from rheumatic heart diseases…be healed from all heart defects**…be healed my good friend from congenital heart diseases…be healed and live well in that healing and saving name of the Lord Jesus Christ. May the God our Father make his children happy in their hearts. May he speak forth joy and happiness. May he supply ways and means that bring healing and gladness to your heart and body. May the good Lord bring restoration to your life that touches your hearts. **May he stop your heart from bleeding**. May he remove tears from your heart. Heart; be healed in the name of the Lord Jesus Christ, be beautiful. Heart, see beauty, you are full of splendour and majesty. Be healed from illness… **Heart; you are brilliantly surrounded with beauty and love. Heart; you are well connected to good veins and arteries**…Heart, receive the good desires of life and be happy. Be healed dear heart…be healed from troubles and struggles…be healthy in the body…**Heart; be refined. Be healthy…be freed from pain. Live!** You are a beautiful heart. Heart; be special; be more than a diamond, be more than a sapphire, be more precious than a ruby, and be above an emerald. You belong to God…you are the temple of the Holy Spirit of God…be healed dear heart…Be precious dear heart…**Heart; be a long lasting precious love of God Almighty.** Heart, be true and faithful to the body. Be durable. Be strong. Be kind. Be full of life and glamour. Be robust dear heart in the name of the Lord Jesus Christ. Heart; know and understand that there is sunshine in your life…there is the beauty of the Lord for your long life…there is more light for you dear heart…there is powerful good healing light for your life…**Be healed dear heart**…be healed in that powerful name of the Lord Jesus Christ.

• **Dear Reader speak out;** speak words of life and say; "I was purchased by the blood of Jesus and I remain obedient because the Spirit of the most supreme God is upon me…My heart was purchased for God…My heart lives for God in every moment…all days…all months…all seasons…all years…Yes…the good and perfect Holy Spirit reigns in my life forever and ever. I have given my heart and life to my God who is Maker of heaven and earth…the healer of my heart."

Deuteronomy 30:6

"The LORD your God will circumcise your hearts and the hearts of your descendants, so that you may love him with all your heart and with all your soul, and live."

* Be healed in your heart…may the Lord God Almighty, whom you love, bless your heart and your children`s hearts in the name of the Lord Jesus Christ. **May he reverse the curse of heart diseases in the family…May the Lord remove the curses of veins and arteries from your body and family…be well in your heart, veins and arteries…be blessed in your veins and arteries…be healed in your body…be immersed in the saving and protecting blood of the Lord Jesus Christ…**May the good Lord in the name of Jesus remove all ill spoken words of heart failure and heart disease…may the Almighty One remove weaknesses of the heart in families and people…May the Almighty One breathe his blessings to the heart…may God Almighty cancel the spirit of curses, bad omens concerning hearts of people…Be healed in your

heart…be protected with the healing presence of God Almighty, Maker of heaven and earth…be healed in the heart…be healed from illness of the heart…be set free from chronic illness of the heart…be healed from pain and struggling of the heart…be immersed in the blood of the Lord Jesus Christ…be healed my good friend…be removed from having a weak heart…be blessed with a strong and healthy heart…be healed in that wonderful name of the Lord Jesus Christ…be healed, you and your family…be protected from the evils of heart attacks and strokes…be healed with healthy hearts…be protected in the heart…Be healed in every part of your heart…Hallelujah! May the good Lord bless your descendants…may his heart dwell upon them…**May he bless them with sound hearts**…be healed in the heart…May there be perfection in your heart…be favoured and strengthened in the heart…May God Almighty bless your genes…you belong to God Almighty…you were perfected on the cross where the Lord Jesus Christ died and saved you from condemnation…He rose and conquered death and the curse of sin for you…you resurrected with Christ…your heart resurrected with Christ…your heart is re-born in righteousness, truthfulness, faithfulness, justice and peace…**you have the right to receive healing and salvation from God Almighty in the powerful and redeeming name of the Lord Jesus Christ…**You have a right to be saved in the wonderful name of the Lord

Jesus Christ…Be healed in the heart my good friend…Be healed in completeness…May the love of God fill your heart and heal you…may the good Spirit of the Lord dwell in your heart and bring favour…your life is protected with the blood of the Lord Jesus Christ.

Jeremiah 17:10

"I the LORD search the heart and examine the mind, to reward a man according to his conduct, according to what his deeds deserve."

* **Be healed from irregular and abnormal arteries**. May the good Lord protect the heart and arteries from all kinds of viruses and undesirable substances. **Be healed from blood clotting diseases…**may the good Lord wipe out blood clotting disorders…**be healed in the heart, arteries and veins**…be well in your veins, arteries and heart…be healed from terminal illness of the heart, veins and arteries…**be protected from the collapse of veins and arteries…**be well in the veins and arteries…be well in your body and heart…be healed through the healing flow of God Almighty, flowing in your heart with a powerful healing…be healed in goodness…be healed in peace…be healed with love and mercy from God Almighty…be healed from illness of the heart…be healed in the name of the Lord Jesus Christ…**Be healed from aneurysm**…May the good Lord protect your arteries and veins from

bursting…May he bring good strength and security…be healed in your veins and arteries in that powerful name of the Lord Jesus Christ…Prosper in the heart…be healed and be protected from heart strokes in that powerful and present name of the Lord Jesus Christ. **May the Lord protect your mind from erosion by giving you a sound heart and a sound flow of blood in your body…Be healed in the blood vessels**…May the Lord give favour to your heart so that you live a long life…May the good Lord, in the powerful name of the Lord Jesus Christ give you a meaningful life through the blessing of a healthy heart…Be healed my good friend…be healed in your heart…may all the pain, tightness and weakness leave your body and heart…breathe in peace in the powerful name of the Lord Jesus Christ. Be able to eat and not get worried about your heart…be able to walk and not grow faint…be able to run and be intact in the heart…be able to be active have a good and healthy heart- bit…**may there be strong balance and health in the heart**…may the Lord Almighty bless your heart with sound healing…May he drive away the spirit of death and decay from your heart…Be strong in the powerful and saving name of the Lord Jesus Christ.

* **Be healed with good strength in your heart**…May the good Lord keep you safe in times troubles, trials and tribulations… do not be misled to evil things and ways. Do not allow fear to overwhelm you…Rise above the

spirit of fear by trusting and declaring strongly in the healing and protecting presence of the Lord Almighty who created you and all heaven and earth and the things that dwell in it…Do not seek the ungodly means of healing and solutions. Remove dirty things from your life…remove the grime and all stains in your life by surrendering your heart to Jesus Christ…Stay with what is pure and healing…Give your whole heart to the one who purifies it…the Lord Jesus Christ…surrender to the Holy Spirit and live in his perfect righteousness and everything will all go well with you…Yeah…stay with Jesus Christ in your hearts and be healed in truth and in spirit. Give complete trust to God and he will heal your disease and break the chains of oppression from this illness. Be steadfast in faith in the healing power found in the redeeming blood of Jesus. God is a faithful God who will give the reward of trusting him. Continue to walk in his light and all will go well with you. Be healed in the heart…be healed in the wonderful and saving name of the Lord Jesus Christ

1John 3:23

"And this is his command: to believe in the name of his Son, Jesus Christ, and to love one another as he commanded us."

* In the name of the Lord Jesus Christ…may the good Lord bless and purify the blood that flow in the veins

and all over the body with good nutrients and good breath and good health… **May the good Lord in his power, iron out all blood diseases from your body.** May there be a good and healthy blood texture required for your body. May your blood count be perfected in the powerful name of the Lord Jesus Christ. May the Lord God Almighty remove all thinning of the blood in your veins…**may the wonderful Lord wipe away all blood clots and restore your blood to perfection…may there good order in your blood, veins and arteries…**may the Lord bless your blood and make it healthy…may he wipe out all disorder in your blood…**be purified in your blood**…be cleansed in completeness in your blood…**be healed in your blood vessels**…be healed in the wonderful name of the Lord Jesus Christ…May the good Lord heal and protect you from the spirit of disease and suffering…may God Almighty remove the spirit of rotting of the blood in your body…may his newness be established in your blood all the days of your life…be healed in your blood…**be healed from HIV/AIDS**…be healed from all viruses that attack your blood…be purified in your blood…be healed from terminal illness of the blood…**be living and active in your blood, veins and arteries…**be healed in your body…be healed from illness…**be healed from chronic illness of the blood, veins and arteries**…be well in your blood , veins and arteries…**be healthy in your blood vessels**…be set free from being controlled by a chronic illness…be saved from living a life with a disease…be healed in your body…be healed in your flesh and blood…be healed from terminal illness of the blood…be healthy in your blood and body…be healed with a complete healing from God Almighty who is Maker of heaven and earth…be healed through his mercy and love…be forgiven from all your sins…be healed in your blood…be healed from HIV/AIDS…be healed, you and your family…be healed you and your spouse…be healed in your bodies…be healed in power…be healed from illness…be healed through the mercy of God Almighty…be blessed with the spirit of righteousness…be holy because God Almighty, who is your God is a holy God…be holy because the Lord Almighty, who forgives your sins, requires you to be holy all the days of your life…be healed with a complete and permanent healing from the Almighty One…Be healed with the wonderful flow of healing from a Mighty God who is all-Powerful and all-Redeeming…be healed in the name of the Lord Jesus Christ, the Lamb of God who took away the sins of the world…**May the Lord God Almighty protect you from meningitis, aneurysm, sepsis, strokes, heart attacks, diarrhea and dehydration.** Be healed in your body… be healed from all forms of illness…be immersed in the saving and protecting blood of the Lord Jesus Christ…Be healed through the powerful healing flow of God Almighty,

Maker of heaven and earth, the Sovereign I AM, the
Holy One, the Good Shepherd of your heart and soul,
the wonderful and caring Shepherd of your life…be
healed in his care and love…be healed in his mercy and
love…be immersed in that saving and protecting blood
of the Lord Jesus Christ, the Lamb of God who took
away the sins of the world…the love of God the Father
for the people he redeemed…**Hallelujah; may the
Lord Almighty, touch your blood and bring
smoothness to it**…may he remove all clots and heal
you…may the Lord bless the veins and arteries that carry
your blood…may he breathe his healing breath in
them…**may the Good Lord heal you from chronic
illness of the blood, veins and arteries**…be healed in
that wonderful name of the Lord Jesus
Christ…Hallelujah. May your heart and mind be in good
peace. Be healed in your blood, body and heart…be
healed with goodness…be healed in that powerful name
of the Lord Jesus Christ, the Lamb of God who took
away the sins of the world…Hallelujah!

* **Dear Reader, pray;** "Father God Almighty…I pray
that you give me a sound mind, a sound heart, sound
blood and sound body of Christ. I surrender to the
Holiness of my King. I surrender my heart to you King
of kings…Lord of Lords…I give you my life because
you are the origin of life itself…you are my heart that
will never perish…you are the Lord and master of my
heart…you are the blood that flows in my veins and

arteries…You are my power than can never be stolen or broken…I surrender to all your ways and commands. May my life reflect your presence in my heart and soul…I belong to you alone…In you my heart will live and my life will be preserved…"

Isaiah 49:1-4

"Before I was born the LORD called me; from my birth he has mention of my name. He made my mouth like a sharpened sword, in the shadow of his hand he hid me; he made me into a polished arrow and concealed me in his quiver. He said to me, "you are my servant, Israel, in whom I will display my splendour." But I said, "I have laboured to no purpose; I have spent my strength in vain and for nothing. Yet what is due me is in the LORD`s hand, and my reward is with God.""

* Heavenly Father…may your will be done in my life. I surrender myself to you…I surrender my heart and soul to you…I surrender my life to Jesus Christ…I surrender all my cares, I surrender all my brokenness, my ambition, my heart feelings of hurt and pain, I surrender all illnesses to you my God and my Father. I surrender all that I am to you my Saviour and the Healer of my life, Jehovah Raphe. I surrender my fears, my past troubles and suffering, I surrender my bruised heart to you…I surrender to your mending of my brokenness…I surrender to your knowledge and understanding. God

knows best because he sees everything and he is
everywhere and he is all powerful. Yes…may the Lord
be in me and with me…I surrender my heart`s wishes
and desires to my Sovereign Lord. I surrender to your
goodness and purpose for my life. I surrender to you,
my life giving God…I surrender to what is true, faithful
and abounding in love. In all humbleness, I surrender
my life to you God Almighty. My surrender my weak
heart to you for I cannot go on without you my Lord
and my Master…I surrender my heart for healing and
salvation…I surrender to God Almighty…I surrender to
the Lord who is enthroned high above for the sake of
his purpose in my life. I surrender to your glory and
honour…I surrender! I Surrender to the healing flow of
God in my heart…I surrender to the healing flow
touching every part of my heart…Flow healing of
God…flow and make my heart strong…flow and use
my heart for your goodness…flow healing flow of God
Almighty…flow in my heart and heal me in your love,
mercy and will…flow wonderful healing of a mighty
God and bring all goodness to my heart…Flow and heal
me Lord…Flow in every part of my heart and bring
steadfast and permanent healing to my heart, body and
mind…Flow and protect me with your healing
flow…Flow healing flow of God…flow and heal me in
completeness…Flow in every cell…flow…flow
wonderful healing of Almighty God…flow in my
heart…flow in every muscle…flow in the aorta…flow in

the ascending aorta an bring goodness to the head and arms…flow in the descending aorta and bring goodness to the lower body…flow in my veins and arteries…flow in all my heart chambers…flow healing flow of God Almighty…Flow and heal every part of my heart and body…Flow in my heart muscles…flow in every heart valve…flow in all muscles…flow in all fibre and tissues and bring powerful healing to my heart…preserve my heart in your healing flow…flow holy healing flow of God Almighty…Flow and bring your wonderful healing to my body and heart…flow and heal my soul…Flow in your healing powerful flow and take control of your heart and body…flow and bring life to my soul…flow healing flow of a wonderful and triumphant God Almighty…flow and rescue my heart from peril…flow and shield my heart from failure…flow and cover me with your mighty protecting flow…flow healing flow of God Almighty…Flow in my heart all the days of my life and heal me with your goodness and love…flow and make my heart good and wonderful…take away all hardness…take away all evil…mend my broken heart with your healing flow…Make me yours in all my ways and feelings…Flow healing flow of God Almighty…Heal me for I belong to you…my body and heart is the temple of your Holy Spirit…Flow healing flow of God and heal me with your permanent and true healing…bring sweet healing to my heart and body…I surrender to your healing flow…I surrender to your

Sovereign Healing flow healing my heart and body and mind...I ask all this in the wonderful name of the Lord Jesus Christ...I surrender to your healing flow in that powerful and saving name of the Lord Jesus Christ!

Psalm 119: 76-77

"May your unfailing love be my comfort, according to your promise to your servant. Let your compassion come to me that I may live, for your law is my delight."

* May the love of God flow in your veins...may his compassion fill your heart...Be healed from all blood diseases...**be healed from Leukemia...may the blood flow in your veins peacefully and healthily**...be purified in veins, arteries and the blood that flow in them...**be healed from terminal illness of the blood, veins and arteries...**be healed in that wonderful name of the Lord Jesus Christ...May the good Lord breathe in life in your bowels...be healed in your metabolism...be healed in the name of the Lord Jesus Christ...**May the Lord Almighty, in the name of the Lord Jesus Christ bless your intestines with stability and favour**...May the good Lord heal your from trauma...may the good Lord remove all disturbances from your life...be healed from pain and suffering...be stable in the heart and mind...be healed in all his goodness...be healed my good friend from the top of your head to the soles of your feet. May God Almighty remove the ordeal, stress

and shock brought by illness…May the good Lord in his compassion wipe away this disease in the wonderful and comforting name of the Lord Jesus Christ…May the healing flow of God move strongly in your blood and blood cells and bring healing to your body…be strong and healthy in your blood…may the breath of the Lord be present in your blood…be healed in the powerful name of the Lord Jesus Christ. Live…be strong…do not be weak…do not be dizzy…have good balance in your body and mind…be healed in completeness in that wonderful name of the Lord Jesus Christ.

* **Dear Reader,** speak to the Holy God and say; "Lord, my heart is for you alone…there is no other besides you. Heal me through your compassion. Protect my heart from demise…make my heart and body strong…Heal me Lord…heal my heart with your good and powerful permanent strength…Pour your love upon my heart and life…bless me with your breath of healing…Keep my heart safe and sound in your loving care…Be the good Shepherd of my heart and life…Heal me Lord for I belong to you…heal my heart with your divine presence…Overcome all illness of the heart…help me Lord, I am your child…Let me live in your name and in your good presence all the days of my life in this land of the living…Let my life be a testimony of your love and glory. Lord, help me and lift me up. Take away all my fear and insecurity in my life. Take away all illness of the heart and body…Protect me all the days of my

life…protect me in your glory…heal my heart with a permanent healing flow…Remove all heart attacks…save my heart from failing…heal me in the name of the Lord Jesus Christ…Give me stability and relief from all trials of this life."

Luke 9:58

"Jesus replied, "Foxes have holes and birds of the air have nests, but the Son of Man has no place to lay his head."

* May the power and presence of the Lord keep you safe…May the good lord bring stability in your body and heart…Be healed from weakness and numbness. May the Lord remove all confusion from your life and body. Be healed from headaches…may the blood carry good oxygen to your brain…have enough oxygen in your brain and live…be strong in the brain…May the Lord bless your veins and brain with a strong and unshakeable protection…**May he bless your mind with a strong and long lasting memory**. May he help you to remember and recollect your past and near, far and present memories…be alert…grasp meaning to the things in your life…be healed my good friend…May the good Lord be in good control of your health and body…May he give you ability to move…May the good Lord keep you from going under…rise up…be healed in his power…be stable…be diligent…be able…have

strength…have good balance and body coordination…have perfect and good sound vision…be healed in the glorious and healing name of the Lord Jesus Christ…Yes be healed my good friend…be healed in that saving name above every name…the name of the Lord Jesus Christ.

* **Dear Reader;** speak and surrender to the power of the living God, say; "I surrender all my health, my life…I surrender all my fears…I surrender all my troubles and burdens…I surrender all my worldly gains and pursuits, I surrender them all to Jesus Christ…He has meaning to my life…he has given me life in my heart and veins…he has given strength and goodness in my heart…I surrender to Jesus, I surrender to the Kingdom of God…I give all my life to Jesus Christ my Saviour…I have regained my strength in his name…I do what Jesus wants me to do all the days of my life and I know God my Father will heal me in completeness and fill me up according to his mercy and love through Jesus Christ my Saviour and King. I give my heart to Jesus Christ my redeemer."

Proverbs 15:30

"A cheerful look brings joy to the heart, and good news gives health to the bones."

* Be healed in your heart…be healed in your body…be healed in your brain…**be healed in your bones and marrow**…be healed from bone marrow cancer…be completely healed in the name of the Lord Jesus Christ…Be healed in your life…be filled with joy and happiness…be surrounded with goodness that speak well to your heart…**be completely strong in the heart**…be able to endure in the heart…be healed and be set free from the spirit of torment…be happy in the name of the Lord Jesus Christ…Be set free from the spirit of grief…be filled with the goodness from God Almighty who is mighty to save and to protect…Be able to endure…be able to tolerate and live in goodness…be happy in the heart…be hopeful in your heart…be healed in the name of the Lord Jesus Christ…**Rise above in the heart**…be steadfast in the saving power of the Lord…be upright in your heart…Hallelujah; be completely healed in your heart all the days of your life in that wonderful name that is above every name…be healed…be healed with a wonderful healing from God Almighty…be healed in strength…be healed with peace in your veins and arteries…be healed with peace in your heart…be healed in that wonderful and prevailing name of the Lord Jesus Christ….be healed….

Zechariah 10:6-8

"I will strengthen the house of Judah and save the house of Joseph. I will restore them because I have compassion on them. They will be as though I have not rejected them; for I am the LORD their God and I will answer them. The Ephraimites will become like mighty men, and their hearts will be glad as with wine. Their children will see it and be joyful; their hearts will rejoice in the LORD. I will signal for them and gather them in. Surely I will redeem them; they will be as numerous as before."

* Be healed and protected from brain damage...Come forth...Be healed from the top of your head to the soles of your feet. Be strong again. May the good Lord be the command of everything you do...all your thinking...may he reside in all your senses and perfect them...May he be in your speech...may he direct you charismatic voice...may he be present in all that you say and do...Breathe in his name...speak, do not mumble...do not groan...be healed in your nerves...Be able to breathe...have ability to move your muscles and swallow your food and saliva...**Do not drool**...be healed in all your motor skills...be healed in all your muscles...be healed from the stronghold of paralysis...be healed in power in your body...be revived in your body...have good and healthy feelings in your body...be restored with a wonderful good sense of touch and movement in your body...be healed in the name of the Lord Jesus Christ...**Move your body...move your eyes**...have a good bowel movement...be able in the power of the Lord Almighty...Rise up...be healed in his glorious name...In the name of the Lord Jesus Christ, live

again…be completely healthy in body, soul and spirit…**be healed in every cell, in every fibre, joints and marrow and in every tissue in your body**…be healed in your bones…be restored to goodness…be revived in your body… be whole and multiply in the power of the Lord who created heaven and earth. Be happy and be fearless. Be blessed with a long and happy fruitful life. Be healed in the name of the Lord Jesus Christ.

Proverbs 19:21

"Many are the plans in a man`s heart, but it is the LORD`s purpose that prevail."

* Be healed from stroke…recover…have balance, have sound coordination in the body…have strong muscles…have strong fibre tissues…be firm and sound in body…Do not shake…do not be clumsy…be healed in your brain and be healed in your body movement…be healed in the heart and arteries…be healed my good friend…you will be healthy again…you will walk and run again…**you will be able to take care of your personal body and life…You are blessed**…you are loved…the Lord will make you well again…be healed in the powerful and conquering name of the Lord Jesus Christ…Heart disease is conquered in the name of the Lord Jesus Christ…heart stroke is prohibited from coming into your life once and for all in the name above

every name…heart attack is demolished and conquered in the protecting name of the Lord Jesus Christ and the power in the blood of the Lord Jesus Christ which never fails…Be healed in his righteous and holy name

* **Dear Reader in Christ**, be in agreement; "Hallelujah: I am healed through God`s mercy and will. I am healed in the blood of the Lord Jesus Christ my Saviour and King."

2Thessalonian3:3

"But the Lord is faithful, and he will strengthen and protect you from the evil one."

* "Why should I be afraid? I belong to a powerful God who is mighty to save and to protect…I belong to a righteous God Almighty. He demolishes false thrones in my life, he brings justice and peace. He fights for my life…He heals me…He heals my heart. He mends my brokenness. He declares life for me and for my sake he rises up to help and conquer. I believe therefore I hope in him alone. I stand strong in his care. **Nothing will pull me down…the Lord Almighty protects me…the Sovereign I AM, the Holy Spirit, intercedes on my behalf for the sake of my life and for the sake of his name…He takes away the grave from the path of my life…he removes all brokenness and hopelessness…the Lord keeps my light burning, he**

preserves my life in his goodness…he keeps my life going…disease is defeated. Fear is removed…loneliness is destroyed…restlessness is demolished and I am bestowed with the strength that come from God Almighty in the name of my Lord Jesus Christ. All trials in my life are calmed down and I feel his strong protecting presence in my life. I belong to Jesus Christ my Saviour."

Colossians 2:2-3

"My purpose is that they may be encouraged in heart and united in love, so that they may have the full riches of complete understanding in order that they may know the mystery of God, namely, Christ, in whom are hidden all the treasures of wisdom and knowledge."

* Lord Jesus Christ…stay in my heart forever and ever. You are the Lord of my life…the Master of my soul. My heart knows you alone.

Psalm 28:7

"The LORD is my strength and my shield; my heart trusts in him, and I am helped. My heart leaps for joy and I will give thanks to him in song."

* Be set free from bondage and sadness…**God's heart is for you**…his sacred heart bring protection to your

heart…his sacred heart carries your soul…be healed in the heart…May the good heart transport blood in goodness and sacredness…be healed my good friend…be healed in the heart…**May the joy of the Lord reside in your heart, veins and arteries**…may his beautiful healing flow pass through your heart veins and all arteries…yes…may his powerful heart convey love to your life… be healed in your heart, veins and arteries…be healed all the days of your life…**stay healthy in your heart, veins and arteries…**be blessed with longevity in your heart, veins and arteries…be healed in the name of the Lord Jesus Christ…

Psalm 31:14-15

"But I trust in you, O LORD; I say, "You are my God." My times are in your hands; deliver me from my enemies and from those who pursue me.""

* Be freed from all suffering, may the good Lord touch all the pressing issues and all trials from the bottom of your heart all the way up in the Name of Jesus. May he remove sadness and discontentment. May he fulfill his promises in your life in his good name and make you happy in the heart. **Be healed in thy precious heart**. Live in peace and security. May the Lord comfort you in the heart. May he show compassion to the desires of your heart. May the good Lord give you meaningful strength to your heart. May he enable you to live in his

visible and truthful healing ways in your life. Be healed in the name of the Lord Jesus Christ.

Romans 15:13

"May the God of hope fill you with all joy and peace as you trust, so that you may overflow with hope by the power of the Holy Spirit."

* Be healed in your heart, may the good Lord touch all your veins and arteries and bring strength. May the blood in your veins move smoothly…**In the name of Jesus, may the Lord God Almighty unblock all those places blocked in your veins and arteries.** May he remove masses and fat deposits and protect your veins from this attack. **May he create an easy flow of your blood in your veins and arteries…. May he bless your blood.** May the good Lord heal you from terminal illness of the blood…may he protect you from the macabre spirit of rare diseases of the heart and blood…**be healed from rare diseases of the veins and arteries…**May our God Almighty heal your heart from chronic illness…May the Lord surround your heart with his goodness and happiness. Be healed in the heart in the powerful name of the Lord Jesus Christ. Succeed…overcome and be set free…be healed in that powerful and saving name of the Lord Jesus Christ….May the Lord protect your heart with goodness all the days of your life…**may he make your veins and**

arteries clean and strong…may the Lord Almighty heal you with a permanent healing in your veins and arteries…be healed my good friend…be healed with a wonderful and complete healing from God our Father in the name of his Precious Son Jesus Christ…**Be healed with a holy and sacred healing in your vital heart, veins and arteries**…be healed in that innermost being in your body…be healed with a good and happy heart…be healed with wonderful and healthy veins and arteries…be healed in that wonderful name of the Lord Jesus Christ.

Hallelujah.

Thank you Holy Spirit, you are God and you are good all the time.

<u>Bibliography</u>

Powered by the Finger of God, Holy Spirit, Living and Active.

Holy Bible NIV

Good News Bible (American Bible Society)

Bibliography

Powered by the finger of God, Holy Spirit, Living and Active.

Holy Bible NIV

Good News Bible (American Bible Society)